Top 10 professional tips for healthy, natural hair

Sandra Brown

Copyright

Top 10 professional tips for healthy, natural hair

©Copyright 2018 by Author Sandra Brown

Author Sandra Brown
nikkibrown30@yahoo.com

Contents

Introduction

I love my natural hair! Most importantly, I love that I have healthy and low –maintenance hair.

When I was growing up, healthy hair wasn't a major factor when we discussed hair. We all wanted cute hairstyles, but no one cared about healthy hair. That all changed in my late teen years. I fell in love with hair, so I begin to study my hair and focus on keeping it as healthy as possible. My hair was relaxed but also healthy.

I can't recall anyone being concerned about split ends, chemicals in relaxers, or the proper use of flat irons/ curling irons. My hair was relaxed for many years, because we all wanted bone straight hair. No one wanted wavy, curly, or kinky hair.

Does this sound familiar to you? I've maintained my natural hair for almost 6 years, and I want to help you do the same. Do you really want healthy, natural hair? Will you be willing to change your diet for it? Do you know your hair porosity? Will natural hair fit into your daily lifestyle? If so, let me help you along the way. Each chapter will give you a short, detailed tip on how to maintain healthy hair. Enjoy the journey, and love your hair.

Sandra Brown

1

Definitions

Hair Porosityporosity- This refers to your hair's ability to absorb and retain moisture.

High Porosityporosity hair- Hair dries quickly, tangles easily, looks dry and dull and absorbs a lot of moisture.

Low porosity- Hair takes long to dry, doesn't absorb hair color easily, products sit on hair, cuticles are closed, and moisture does not enter easily.

Normal- Absorbs and retains the perfect amount of moisture, always looks healthy and shiny.

Hair shaft- The visible part of the hair that protrudes

through the skin.

It is composed of three layers.

Hair cuticle- The outermost part of the hair shaft.

Cortex- Provides its strength and determines both the color and the texture of the hair.

Medulla- Nearly invisible layer and serves as the marrow of the hair.

Hair density- Your hair density is basically how many strands cover your scalp.

Hair elasticity- This determines how much the hair will stretch and return to its normal state.

Co-wash- Washing your hair with conditioner only. This will add lots of moisture to your hair.

Seal- Moisturize and seal is very important for your hair, and this should be done nightly. Sealing your ends will lock in the moisture to prevent breakage.

2

Best foods for healthy hair

Healthy hair begins with a healthy diet. If you're healthy on the inside, it will radiate on the outside.

I consume a lot of turkey, chicken, avocado, and eggs. These are packed with lots of protein. Protein in your diet helps the body to produce keratin. Your hair is made of mostly keratin.

My absolute favorite is salmon, another amazing source of protein, and it's also full of omega 3 fatty acids, which is essential for our bodies, and we can't produce it on our own.

Again, protein is extremely important in your diet. A lack of protein can force your hair into resting phase, causing older hair to fall out. I eat salmon at least three times a week.

Oysters are also great; you are really missing out if you're not eating them.

They are very high in zinc. Zinc is very essential for growing longer, thicker hair.

If you're not a fan of oysters, beef and lamb are great as well.

Cucumbers are packed with vitamins A, C, and silica. This will improve the elasticity of your hair, also makes it stronger from the inside out and prevents hair breakage.

Citrus fruits are delicious and popular for vitamin C, but red bell peppers have the highest amount of vitamin C, which is highly important for hair growth. Greek yogurt is another great source of protein,; it contains lots of protein and vitamin B5, which helps with blood flow to your scalp. Cinnamon is also essential for healthy hair,; it increases blood flow also. Take a half of teaspoon of cinnamon daily.

Personally, I love spinach and kale. Both are loaded with vitamins A, C, and iron., which helps the red blood cells carry oxygen to hair follicles, which is very essential for healthy hair. These delicious greens will keep your hair moisturized and strong. Last but certainly not least, —water, water, and more water. Drink at least a gallon a day. Water can help with dry scalp and thinning hair, so drink up!

What is my hair texture?

If your hair strand is thin and damages easily, its it's considered to be fine hair.
Medium hair is neither small ornor big, not likely to be damaged.

Coarse hair has a circumference that is wide and thick, and it's not easily damaged. Each of these hair textures can be natural and healthy, when properly taken care of.

What is my Hair Elasticity?

How much can your hair stretch? When healthy hair is wet, it will stretch up to 50% of its original length without breaking.

Low elasticity hair is very susceptible to breakage and hard to curl.

Normal or high elasticity hair is less likely to break and styles easily. If you're unsure of your elasticity, perform this strand test. :

Select four strands of hair from different areas of your head. Make sure the hair is wet,. Hold the hair tightly and stretch the hair. If the hair stretches and returns to its original length when released, then it has good elasticity. If the hair breaks or doesn't return to its original length, you have low elasticity.

What is my Hair Density?

Your hair density can be determined by looking at your scalp to see how much scalp you see.
You can have thick, medium, or thin density.

If it is thick, you won't see any scalp. Medium density, you may see a little scalp, while thin, you will be able to see a lot of scalp. My hair density is thick. You can only see my scalp if it's parted or styled in a way to reveal my scalp.

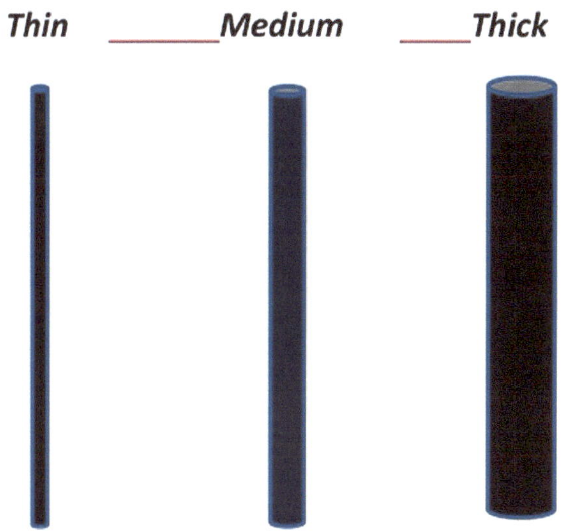
Thin   Medium   Thick

Sandra Brown

3

Hair Test

Daily and weekly hair maintenance

Low manipulation is a major key to having healthy hair. The less styling to your hair means stronger and healthier hair. Healthy hair begins on the inside. Are you working out, meditating, fasting, or praying? Some or all of these should be implemented in your daily and weekly routines. Exercise and fasting can play a major role in your physical health, while meditation and prayer will help you tremendously mentally.

During the colder months, I wear my wigs, braids, or twist outs. Nightly maintenance for my hair includes, moisturizing my ends and sealing in the moisture with coconut oil.

Sweet almond oil or black castor oil is best used if you're experiencing any kind of thinning to your edges or any areas of your scalp. Massaging black castor oil or peppermint oil to your scalp every night before bed will do wonders for your hair.

Peppermint oil and black castor oil can help stimulate hair growth, because of its ability to increase blood circulation to the scalp. The health of my natural hair has been successful because of continuously co-washing. This is when you only apply conditioner to your hair, beginning at the ends of your hair and working your way up to ensure the older hair receives the most moisture, especially if you have normal or high porosity hair.

I have high porosity hair, so I co-wash or shampoo my hair at least twice a week. I usually perform a hot oil treatment and deep condition twice a month.

My hair is shampooed twice with warm water to open my cuticles. First with a deep cleansing shampoo and afterward with a moisturizing or detangling shampoo followed by a 30-minute deep conditioner, covered with a plastic cap.

I also wear a satin bonnet to bed every night. The satin bonnet will protect your hair from drying out, and rubbing against your pillowcase, which can cause breakage.

This will assist with your healthy hair journey tremendously. The average rate for hair .

When styling my hair in the hotter months, I usually leave my hair hanging. Styling my hair up in a scarf is another option, and I only apply gel to the edges of my hair and a light moisturizer throughout my hair. Please don't get caught up in the 'hair type' hype. In my opinion, this is just a marketing scheme for companies to sell products, but knowing your porosity and texture is very important. I promise this will prevent you from wasting money on a lot of unnecessary product.

A few low-maintenance protective styles that I like are: twist outs, braids, and wigs.

The number one way to reduce breakage on your hair is to adopt a low manipulation hair care regimen.

4

Products And Healthy Hair Tips

1. Design essential honey creme moisture retention shampoo, or oat protein & henna shampoo.

2. Design essential almond avocado moisturizing & detangling shampoo .

3. Giovanni tea tree triple treat shampoo for dry and itchy scalp A mixture of apple cider vinegar and water sprayed on my hair and massaged in my scalp for 30 minutes and then shampooed out, relieves dry and itchy scalp as well. Hot oil treatments should be done when hair appears dry and brittle.

4. A mixture of olive oil, sweet almond oil, jojoba

oil, or coconut oil should be warmed to a safe temperature for you and applied to clean hair and covered with a plastic cap for 20 to 30 minutes. Rinse properly and style hair.

5. Giovanni smooth as silk deep conditioner, design essential almond and avocado detangling leave -in conditioner.

6. Design essential almond express moisturizing conditioner Uncle funky's daughter curly magic

7. Carol's daughter black vanilla leave -in conditioner.

8. Carol's daughter hair milk leave- in conditioner.

9. Carol's daughter black vanilla moisture and shine sheen.

Top 10 professional tips for healthy, natural hair

Hot Water vs. Cold Water

Causes frizzy hair	*Frizz-free hair*
Hair is brittle and dry	Seals in moisture
Removes dirt, oil, and build up	Hair is soft and smooth
Opens cuticle	Closes cuticle
Strips hair of natural oils	*Increases shine*

Conclusion

Consistency is the most important factor when it comes to growing and maintaining healthy hair. Natural hair is very easy to maintain, and my haircare tips are based on a comprehensive blueprint for a successful healthy hair journey.

The tips that I'm sharing with you are based on my years of studying and researching various cosmetology books and scientific methods. Most of my tips have been used on my clients throughout their natural hair journey and witnessing tremendous results.

Pretty much like most things in life,

balance is a key factor, and we will never know what works for our hair until we try it. All of my tips may work for one group or most, but remember, whatever you do, it requires balance to discover what works best for your hair.

You may need a little more moisture, while someone else may need less moisture.

Focus on the areas that you need the most improvement, and you should see major improvements. Although, honestly you can try a million products, tips, and foods but one major key to healthy hair is selflove.

Learn to love yourself mentally and physically, and I promise you will see the results you want in all areas of your life. So if having healthy hair is your goal, let the journey begin! Love and blessings to you all.

About the Author

First of all, I would like to thank you for purchasing my book. I truly believe if you follow my tips, you will see the results you desire.

I'm Sandra Brown, a licensed Cosmetologist in Texas and Louisiana. I'm currently a hairstylist in Houston, TX. If you have any questions, please contact me at nikkibrown30@yahoo.com.

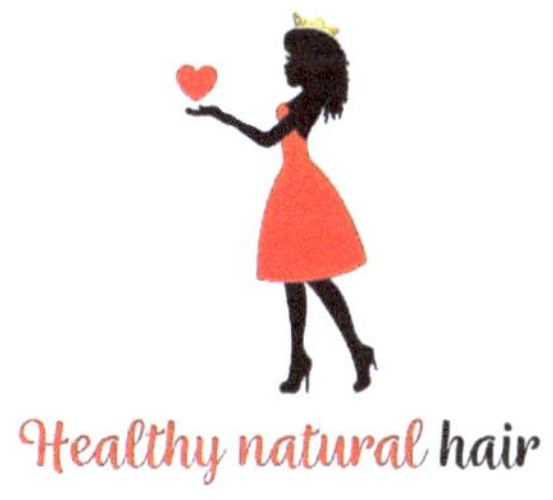

* 9 7 8 1 7 2 0 6 2 6 5 0 3 *